Easy Pregnancy Recipes

Get Your Daily Dose of Nutrition
While Expecting

BY

Rachael Rayner

License Notes

No part of this Book can be reproduced in any form or by any means including print, electronic, scanning or photocopying unless prior permission is granted by the author.

All ideas, suggestions and guidelines mentioned here are written for informative purposes. While the author has taken every possible step to ensure accuracy, all readers are advised to follow information at their own risk. The author cannot be held responsible for personal and/or commercial damages in case of misinterpreting and misunderstanding any part of this Book

Table of Contents

Introduction

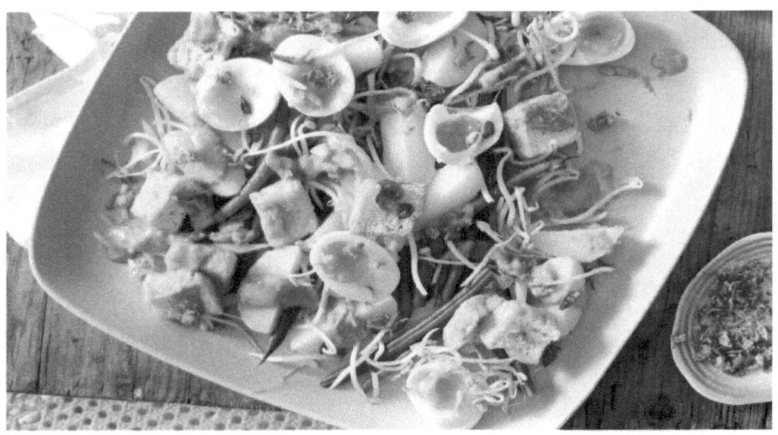

A pregnant woman does not only eat for herself, she needs to worry about her little one too. When a pregnant woman does not eat proper balanced food, they face problems like gas, gestational diseases, high pressure, low pressure, diabetes and constipation. Constipation and gas problem is something every mother faces during their pregnancy. Some even face vomiting which is trigger by different type of food they consume. Not every woman gets vomiting tendency during pregnancy. If you know which ingredient is making you vomit, it is advised to avoid that ingredient.

During pregnancy, a woman should consume good fat like avocado, coconut, almonds, olive oil, and fish. Fish is a very good source of omega 3. Salmon is the number 1 choice for most people. Good veggies like broccoli, cabbage, carrot, pumpkin, potato, cauliflower, asparagus, zucchini, bell pepper, tomatoes and cucumber is good too. Dairy is important for calcium purposes. If you cannot eat dairy, switch to yogurt, sour cream, cheese as they are high in calcium too. Fruits like mango, coconut, kiwi, berries, and peach are good during pregnancy.

This book is designed around food that should be eaten during pregnancy. You will find 30 fabulous smoothies, breakfast, lunches, soups, and even some sweet treats.

Yogurt with Fruits

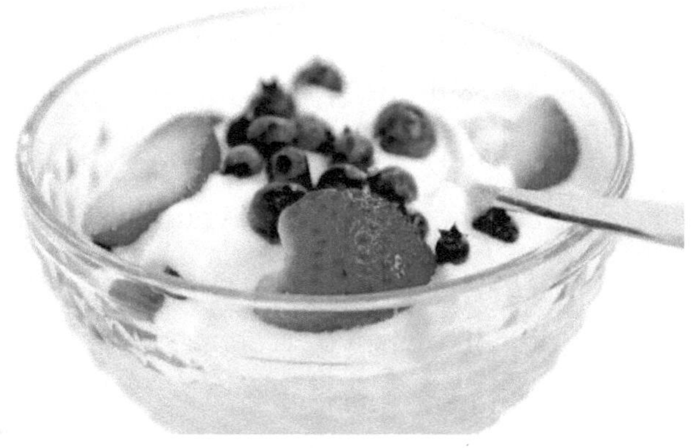

Yogurt is very good for the skin, body and digestion. It is filled with nutrition too. Try to add yogurt in your everyday diet while you are expecting.

Serving Size: 1

Ingredients:

- 1 cup yogurt
- 2 peaches cut into slices
- ½ cup mixed berries
- Fresh mint
- 1 tbsp honey

Instruction:

In a mason jar pour in the yogurt.

Add the fruits and mix.

Add the honey on top. Serve with fresh mint on top.

Sour Yogurt with Apples and nuts

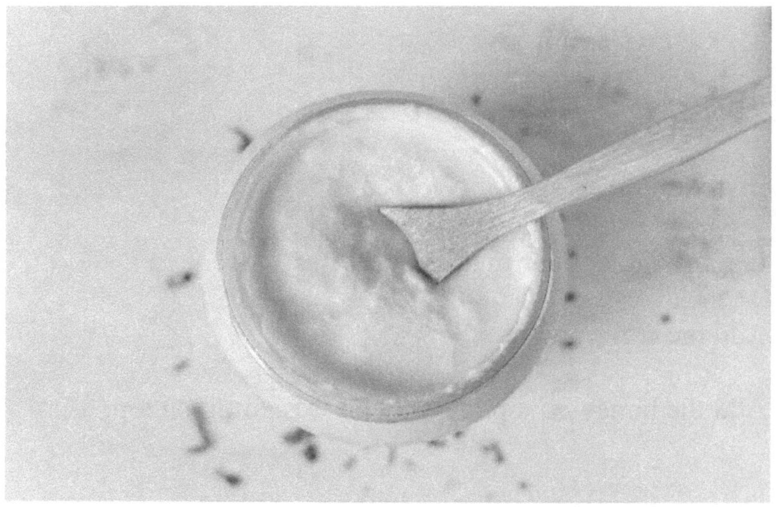

Sour yogurts, nuts and apples, they all complement each other well.

Serving Size: 1

Ingredients:

- 1 cup sour yogurt
- 1 apple
- 2 tbsp chopped pecans
- 2 tbsp chopped pine nuts
- 2 tbsp chopped dates
- A pinch of cinnamon

Instructions:

Cut the apple into small cubes.

In a bowl add the sour yogurt.

Add the apple, dates and nuts.

Add a pinch of cinnamon on top and serve cold.

Date and Nutty Smoothie

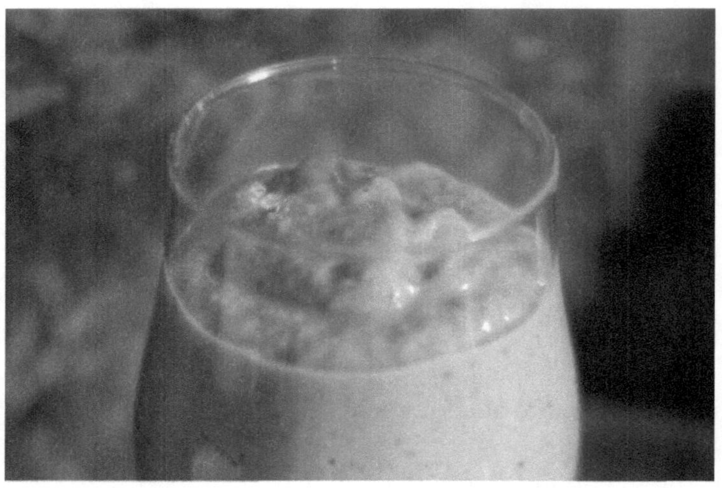

Dates are very good during pregnancy. This is a powerful smoothie that will keep you feeling energetic for hours.

Serving Size: 2

Ingredients:

- 2 cup milk
- ½ cup chopped dates
- ¼ cup nuts of your choice
- Fresh mint

Instructions:

In a blender add the milk with the dates.

Add the nuts and blend until smooth.

Add fresh mint and serve cold.

Yogurt and Strawberry Smoothie

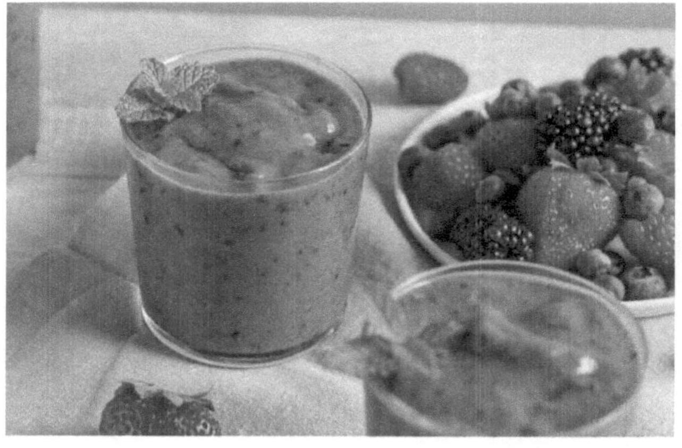

Up your smoothie game by adding yogurt and nuts in it!

Serving Size: 2

Ingredients:

- 2 cup yogurt
- ½ cup diced strawberries
- 5-6 cashews, crushed
- A pinch of salt
- Fresh strawberries to serve

Instructions:

In a blender add the yogurt.

Add the strawberries, cashews and salt.

Blend until smooth. Add fresh strawberries on top and serve cold.

Date and Nut Bars

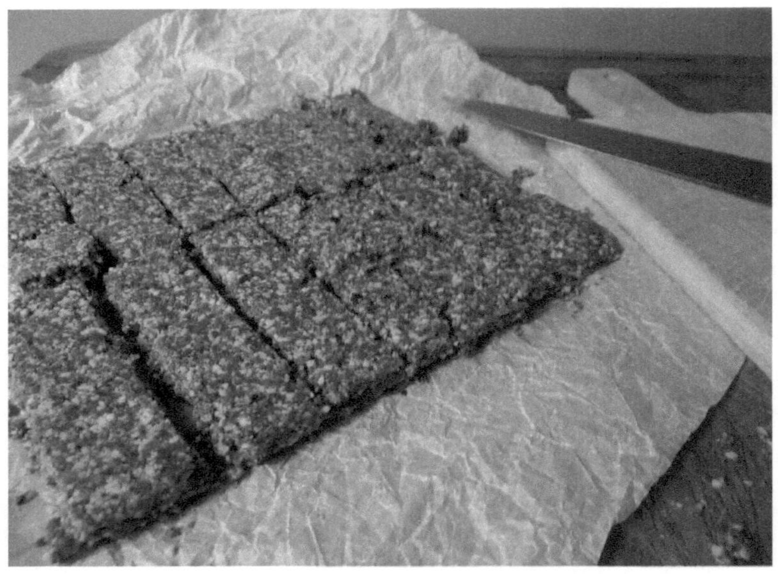

This can serve both as a snack or a dessert. It provides high energy and keep you active for long.

Serving Size: 4

Cooking Time: 5 minutes

Ingredients:

- 2 cup dates
- 1 cup chopped cashew
- ½ cup chopped almond
- A pinch of sea salt

Instructions:

In a double boiler, place the chopped dates and keep stirring until it becomes into a paste.

Take off the heat. Add to a mixing bowl.

Add the salt, nuts and mix using your hands.

Spread on a plane surface and use a knife to cut into squares.

Let it fridge for about 2 hours before serving.

Peanut butter and nut Stuffed Dates

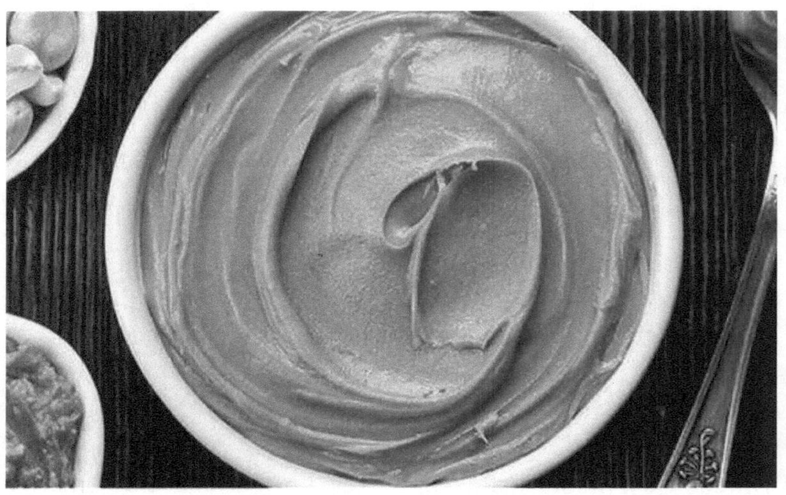

When you want to treat yourself, try this snack.

Serving Size: 4

Ingredients:

- 12-15 dates
- ½ cup pomegranate seeds
- ½ cup peanut butter
- ½ cup yogurt
- Pinch of cinnamon
- ½ cup chopped mix nuts

Instructions:

Make slits on dates and discard the pit.

In a bowl combine the peanut butter, yogurt, nuts and cinnamon.

Stuff the dates using the mix.

Add pomegranate seeds on top and serve.

Healthy Breakfast Muffin

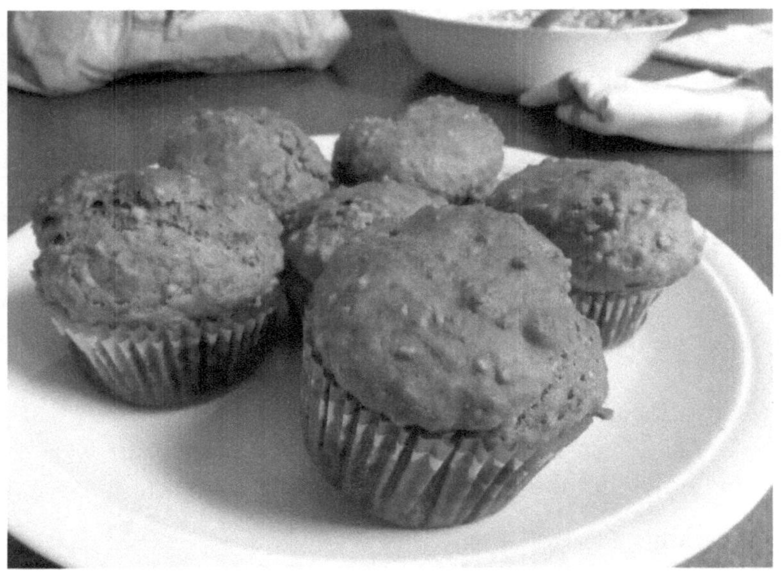

Muffin is amazing at any time of the day. A breakfast is a good little treat you give to yourself.

Serving Size: 20 muffins

Cooking Time: 12 minutes

Ingredients:

- 2 cup flour
- 2 tbsp baking powder
- 2 cup oats
- A pinch of salt
- ½ cup currants
- ½ cup chopped nuts
- 2 eggs
- ½ cup chopped dates
- 1 cup brown sugar
- 1 tsp baking soda

Instructions:

Whisk the eggs in a bowl.

Add the brown sugar and beat until well mixed.

Add the flour, oats, salt, baking powder and baking soda.

Mix gently with a spatula.

Add the nuts, currants and dates.

Mix gently and pour into greases muffin tray.

Bake in the oven for 12 minutes with 350 degrees F.

Serve in room temperature.

Smoked Salmon with Microwave Scrambled Eggs

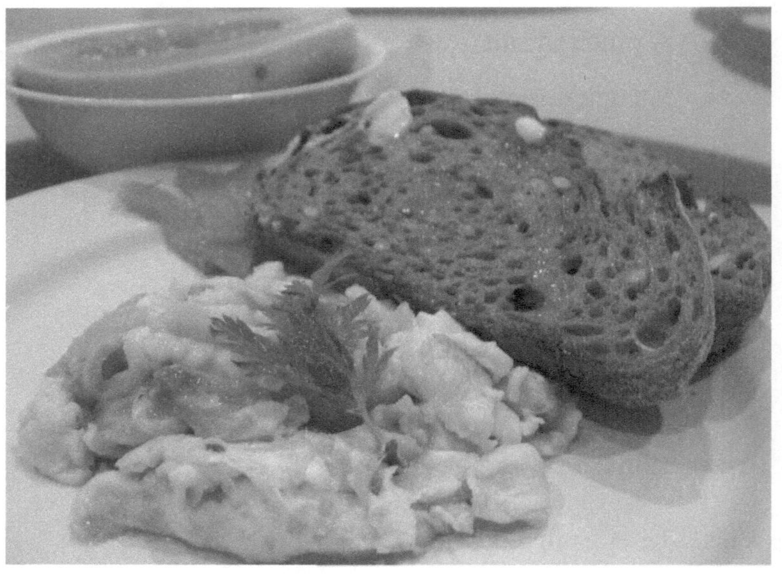

Enjoy a complete balanced breakfast with salmon, egg and bread.

Serving Size: 2

Cooking Time: 8 minutes

Ingredients:

- 2 buns
- 2 eggs
- 1 tsp cold water
- 2 tsp chives, chopped
- 2 oz sliced salmon
- Salt to taste
- Pepper to taste
- 1 tbsp butter

Instructions:

In a bowl add the eggs and mix well.

Add a pinch of salt and pepper.

In a pan, add the butter and heat over medium heat.

Add the egg mix and cook on low heat.

Stir for 2 minutes and transfer onto your buns.

In a grill add the oil and smoke the salmon pieces for 2 minutes.

Add the smoked salmon on top of the eggs.

Add chives, some salt and pepper on top.

Serve.

Cottage Cheese Omelet

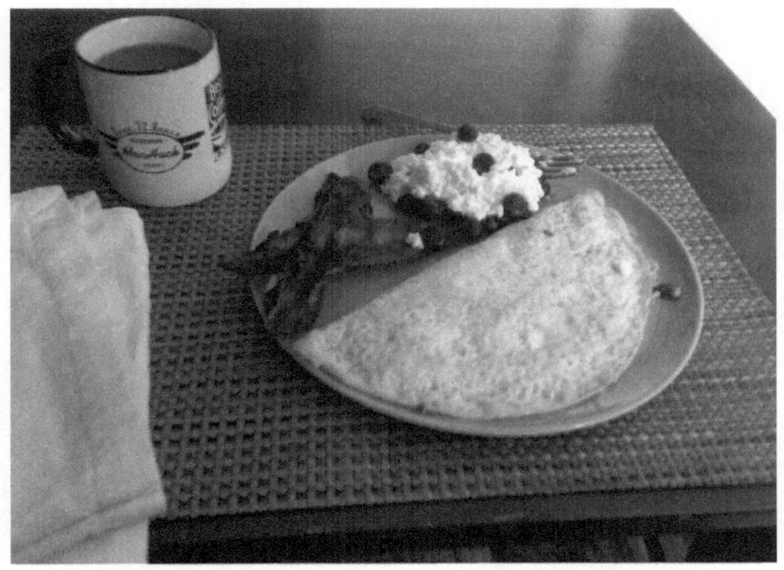

Nothing says breakfast than a finely done omelet!

Serving Size: 1

Cooking Time: 5 minutes

Ingredients:

- 2 eggs
- 1 tbsp olive oil
- 1 tbsp coriander, chopped
- 2 tbsp chopped kale
- Salt to taste
- Pepper to taste
- 1/3 cup cottage cheese
- 4-6 cherry tomatoes cut in half

Instructions:

In a bowl whisk the eggs. Add salt and pepper and mix.

In a pan heat the oil.

Add the egg and cook on medium low heat.

Add the kale, coriander and cherry tomatoes.

Let it cook for 3 minutes and take off the heat.

Add the cottage cheese on top and serve warm.

Fruity Breakfast Cake

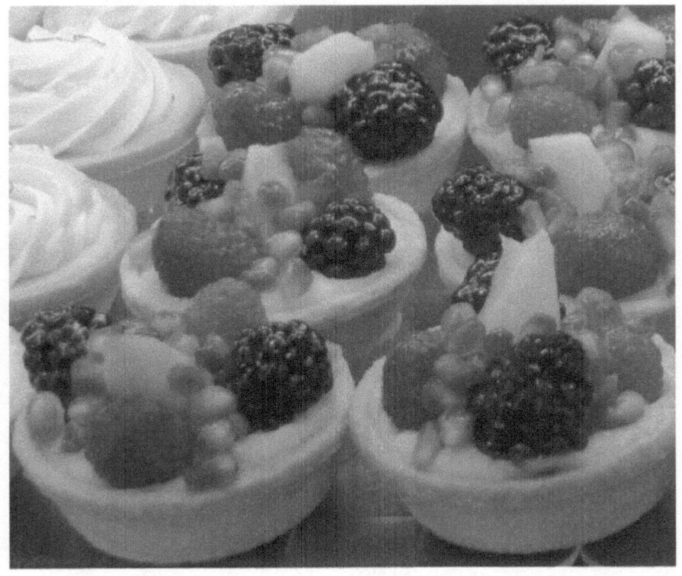

This is not your average cake. This one is definitely on the healthier side yet tastes very good. I have added bunch of nutritious fruits like fig, strawberries, pomegranate into this to boast the health value.

Serving Size: 2

Cooking Time: 10 minutes

Ingredients:

- 2 eggs
- 1 cup Greek yogurt
- 1 cup milk
- 1 tbsp flour
- 1 tbsp brown sugar
- 1 ripe fig, cut into wedges
- 1 banana, mashed
- 1/4 cup pomegranate seeds
- 2 tbsp butter
- 1/4 tsp cinnamon
- 2 tbsp oats
- Strawberries to serve

Instructions:

Whisk the butter with brown sugar.

Add the eggs and beat well.

Add the mashed banana, oats, cinnamon, and flour.

Add the milk and mix well.

Pour into a skillet and bake in the oven for 10 minutes with 400 degrees F.

Add the Greek yogurt, strawberries, pomegranate seeds and figs on top.

Serve in room temperature.

Sweet Breakfast Pie

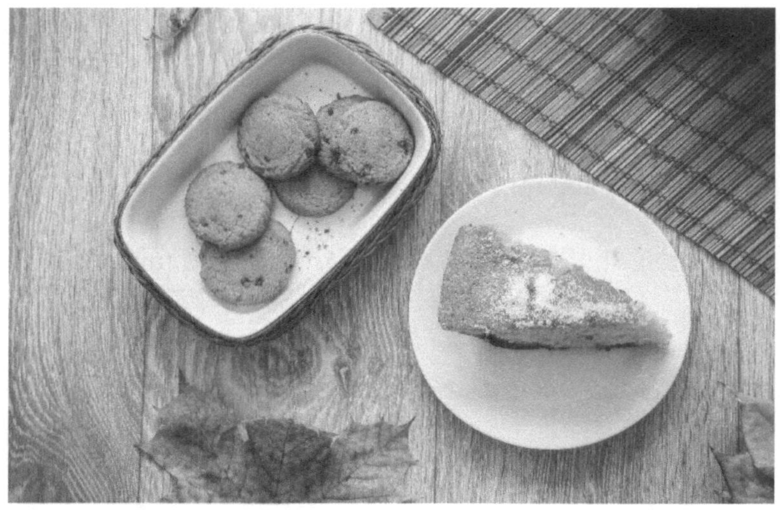

Pies are quite easy to make. They taste good both savory and sweet. This is a sweet breakfast pie recipe with currants, dates and strawberries. You can add your own twist in the same recipe.

Serving Size: 4

Cooking Time: 40 minutes

Ingredients:

- 2 eggs
- 1 tbsp butter
- ½ cup dates, chopped
- 2 tbsp brown sugar
- 1 cup cream
- 2 sheets of puff pastry
- Fresh mint, chopped
- ½ cup currants
- Strawberries to serve

Instructions:

Preheat the oven to 350 degrees F.

Whisk the eggs in a mixing bowl.

Add the cream, butter and sugar. Mix well for 2 minutes.

Add the currants and dates and mix again gently.

Arrange 1 puff pastry onto a baking pan. Add the egg mix onto it.

Add another puff pastry on top. Cut few slits on top to release the air.

Bake in the oven for 40 minutes.

Serve cold or in room temperature with sliced strawberries.

Date pancakes

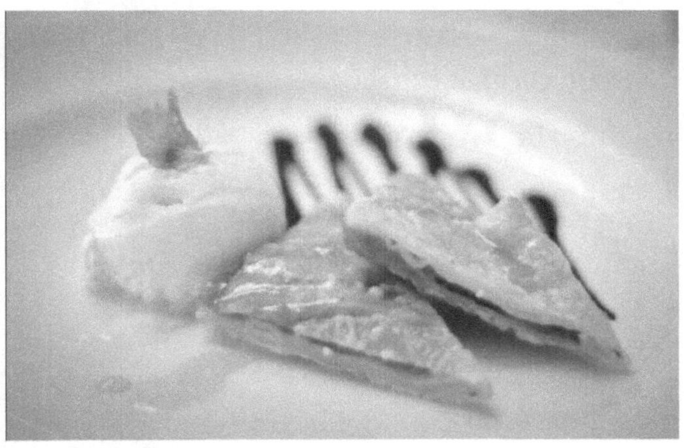

We have tried many pancakes before but nothing tastes as good as date pancakes. Dates are very good for iron, fiber, calcium etc.

Serving Size: 2

Cooking Time: 10 minutes

Ingredients:

- 1 cup flour
- ½ cup date paste
- ¼ tsp coconut extract
- 1 tbsp brown sugar
- 1 tbsp butter
- ½ cup milk
- 1 tsp cinnamon
- A pinch of salt
- 4 tbsp coconut oil

Instructions:

Beat the eggs in a large mixing bowl.

Add the coconut oil, milk, brown sugar and mix well.

Add the coconut extract, and date paste.

Make a smooth mix. Add the salt, cinnamon, flour and mix gently.

Fry them golden brown with butter from both sides.

Serve with more date paste on top.

Papaya Halwa or Papaya Sweet Treats

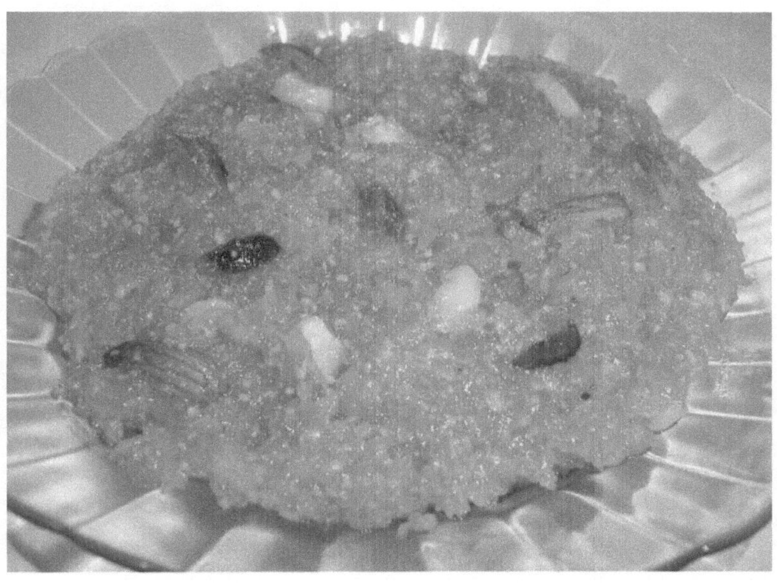

Papaya is very good for digestion and the skin. For a pregnant woman, having proper digestion is very important. This sweet treat can be eaten as a breakfast with tortilla. It can be an evening snack. You can also enjoy it as a dessert at night too.

Serving Size: 2

Cooking Time: 20 minutes

Ingredients:

- 1 raw papaya
- 1 cup milk
- ½ cup cashew, chopped
- 4 tbsp jiggery or brown sugar
- 1 tsp cinnamon
- ½ cup almond, chopped
- 1 tsp cardamom
- A pinch of salt
- 3 tbsp ghee

Instructions:

Peel the papaya and chop it roughly.

Boil them with water until they are very tender.

Drain well and mash using a masher.

In a nonstick pan, add the ghee.

Add the mashed papaya and stir until it gets a slightly darker color.

One by one add all the ingredients.

Keep stirring for 15 minutes straight.

Take off the heat. Spread onto a flat plate.

Use a sharp knife to cut into squares.

Serve cold with more nuts on top.

Green Avocado Coconut Smoothie

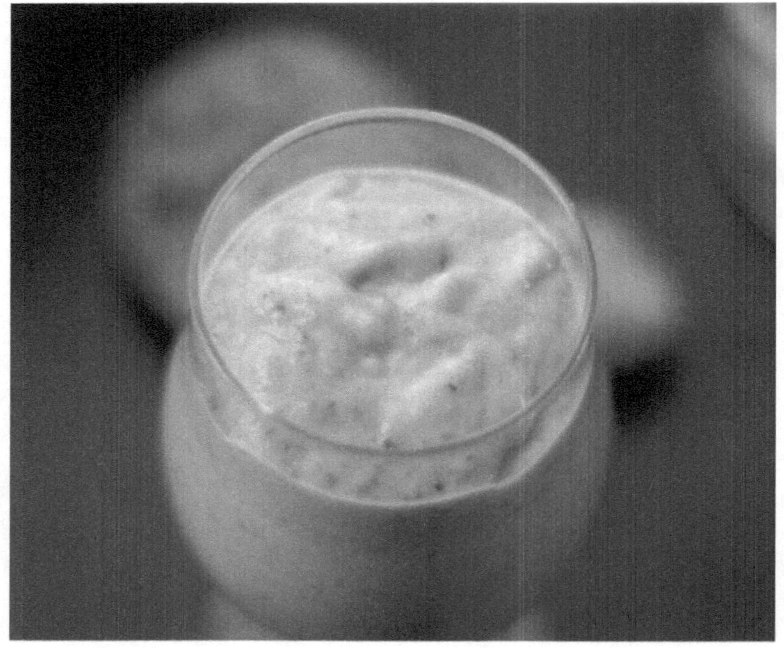

Eating healthy is a good habit every pregnant woman should develop. Start your day with a healthy and tasty smoothie like this one.

Serving Size: 2

Ingredients:

- 2 avocados, cubed
- 2 cup coconut milk
- 6 ice cubes
- 2 tbsp honey
- 1 tsp cinnamon
- Fresh mint
- 1 mango, diced
- ½ cup chopped kale

Instructions:

Add all the fruits into a blender.

Pour in the coconut milk.

Add the honey and blend for 1 minute.

Add the kale, mint, cinnamon and ice cubes.

Blend for another minute.

Serve fresh or cold.

Strawberry Coconut Smoothie

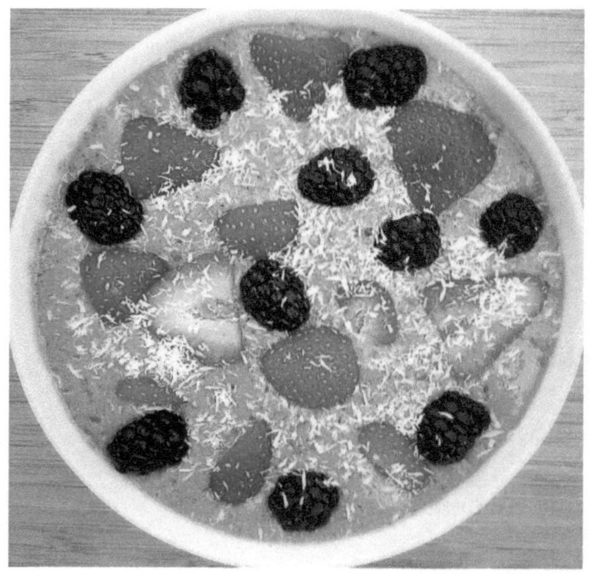

Berries are very good for our health. When you are pregnant, you should munch on these fruits every single day. This smoothie is a great way to boast your energy level and nutrition level.

Serving Size: 2

Ingredients:

- 1 cup strawberries
- 1 cup milk
- 6 currants
- 4 cashews
- 4 almonds
- 6 ice cubes
- 1 tsp cinnamon
- A pinch of salt
- Fresh mint

Instructions:

Add all the fruits in a blender.

Add the milk, salt, mint and cinnamon.

Blend until smooth. Add the ice cubes.

Blend again and serve with mint on top.

Chicken Avocado Tomato Soup

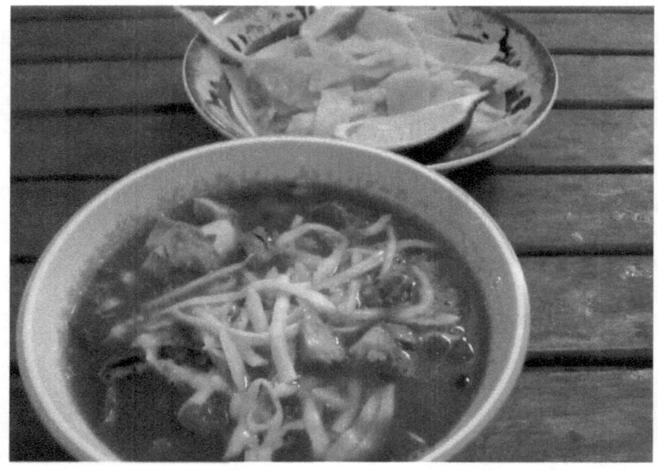

Soup is the ultimate comfort food. It is easy to make. It has many nutritious ingredients like avocado, tomato, chicken and zucchini.

Serving Size: 4

Cooking Time: 30 minutes

Ingredients:

- 4 chicken breasts
- 2 avocados, diced
- 3 tomatoes, diced
- 3 green chilies cut in half
- 1 stalk lemongrass, chopped
- 4 red chilies, whole
- 4 cup chicken broth
- 1 tsp garlic paste
- 2 cup water
- 1 tsp pepper
- 1 tsp cumin
- 1 spring onion, chopped
- Salt to taste
- 2 tbsp olive oil

Instructions:

Add the chicken with broth in a pot.

Let it cook for about 8 minutes.

Transfer the chicken onto a plate and shred it finely.

Return to the pot and add in the rest of the ingredients except the avocado.

Cover with the lid. Let it cook for 20 minutes.

Add avocado and serve hot.

Tropical Fruit Salad

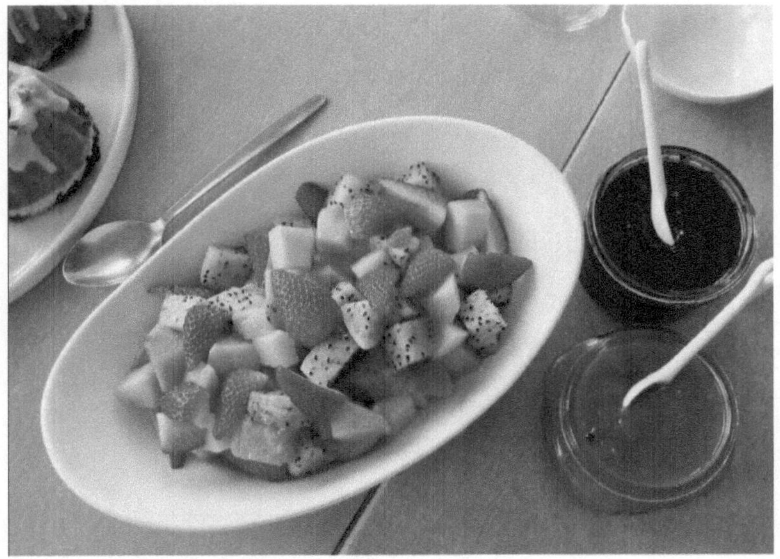

When you are craving for something fresh and fruity, try this salad. The different texture of different types of food makes it really a fun and delightful dish.

Serving Size: 2

Ingredients:

- 2 cucumber, sliced
- 10 cherries
- 2 mangoes, peeled, corded, diced
- 4 avocado, sliced
- 2 onions, chopped
- 2 red chilies, chopped
- 2 tbsp honey
- 1 tsp lemon juice
- 1 tsp pepper
- Salt to taste
- Fresh mint

Instructions:

Toss everything together in a large bowl.

Add honey, lemon juice, salt and pepper.

Serve fresh.

Bean Tomato Soup

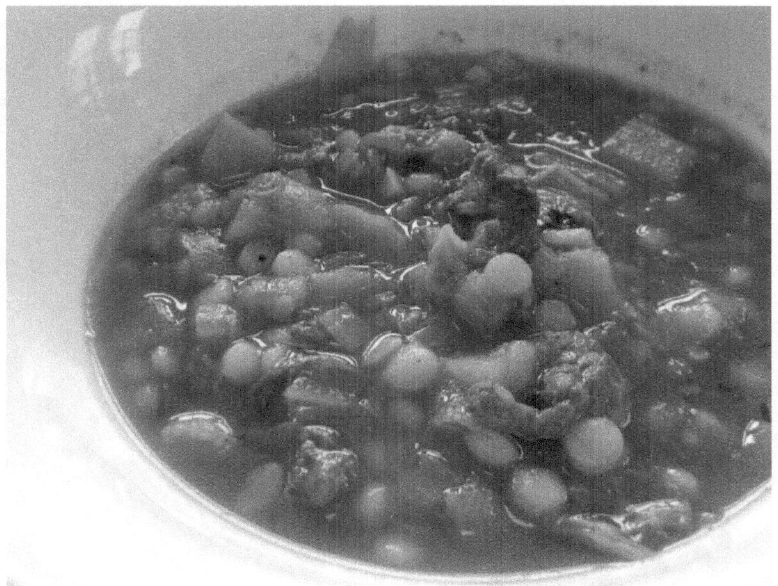

When you know you need to eat something for two and it should keep your energized for long, this is the soup you should make. It contains legume and tomatoes, both are high in carbohydrate and filled with nutrition.

Serving Size: 4

Cooking Time: 2 hours

Ingredients:

- 2 cup white beans
- 1 tbsp vegetable oil
- 1 cup corn kernel
- 2 onion, chopped
- 5 cups vegetable stock
- 2 carrots, diced
- 1 tsp ground cumin
- 1/4 tsp ground black pepper
- 2 tsp chili powder
- 3 garlic cloves, minced
- 1 cup tomatoes, diced
- 2 green chilies
- Fresh coriander
- 2 tbsp tomato paste

Instructions:

Soak the black beans in water for 8 hours or longer.

Wash well and rinse completely.

Add to a pressure cooker with enough water to cover the legumes.

Let it cook for 1 hour with lid on.

Add the rest of the ingredients one by one and cover again.

Cook for another 45 minutes on medium low heat.

Serve hot with fresh coriander on top.

Vegetable and Lentil Stew

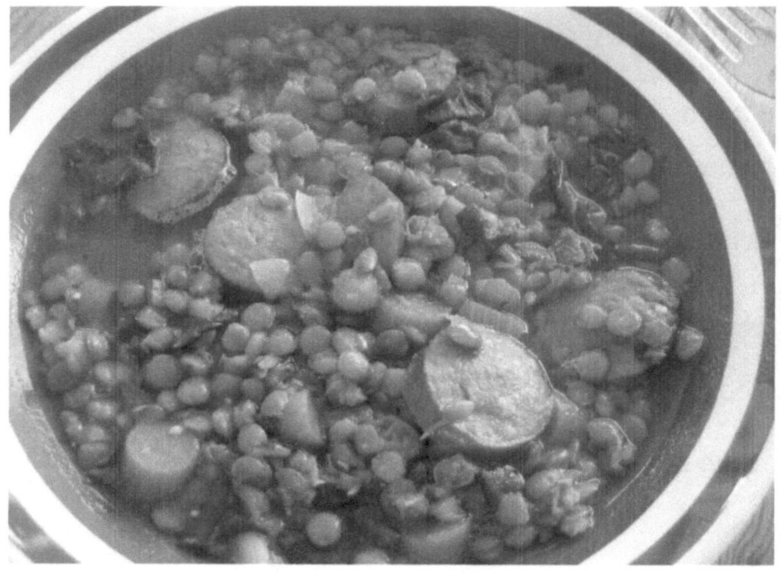

I believe lentil is a great source of protein when you do not want to eat meat. Adding vegetables with a lentil stew elevates the dish by 20%. Serving Size: 4

Cooking Time: 1 hour

Ingredients:

- 1 cup red lentils
- 1 cup chopped onion
- 2 cups shredded cabbage
- 1 cup peeled tomatoes, chopped
- 3 carrots, diced
- 1 tsp mixed herbs
- ½ cup chopped stalk celery
- Salt to taste
- 2 tbsp mustard oil
- 2 cup vegetable broth
- 1 bay leaf
- ¼ tsp black cumin
- 1/4 tsp curry powder

Instructions:

In a pressure cooker heat the mustard oil. Fry the onion golden brown.

Add the black cumin seed and all the spices.

Add 2 tbsp water. Cover and cook for 1 minute.

Add the lentil, stock and cover with lid.

Cook on medium heat for 20 minutes.

Add the vegetables and the remaining ingredients.

Stir well and cover with lid.

Cook for another 20 minutes on medium heat.

Serve hot.

Bean and Pumpkin Stew

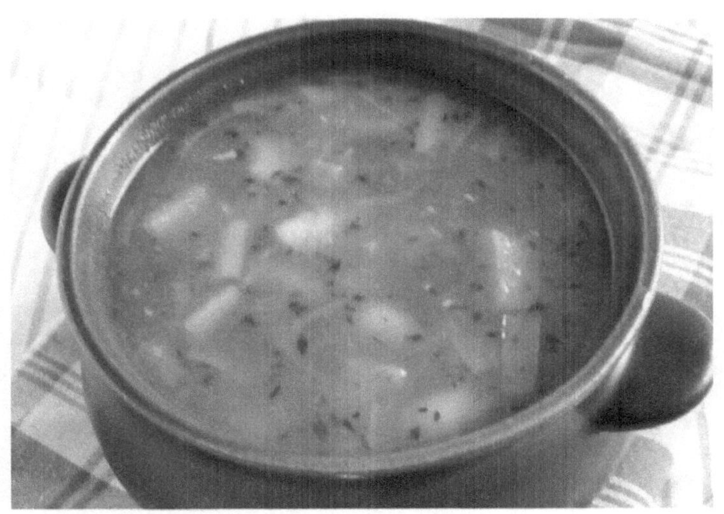

Have you ever tried pumpkin with beans before? They would surprise you how well the final dish turns out! Besides, both pumpkin and beans are very good for a pregnant woman.

Serving Size: 2

Cooking Time: 1 hour

Ingredients:

- 1 cup black beans
- 2 cups vegetable broth
- 1 onion, diced
- 2 cloves garlic, minced
- 1 tsp ground cumin
- Salt and pepper to taste
- 1 cup diced pumpkin
- 1 tbsp olive oil
- 1 tsp soy sauce
- 1 tsp fresh cilantro leaves
- Salt and pepper to taste

Instructions:

In a pressure cooker boil the beans with water for 30 minutes.

Transfer the beans into a bowl.

In a pan heat the oil.

Fry the garlic and onion golden brown.

Add the soy sauce, cumin, and pumpkin.

Toss for a minute and add the beans.

Add the broth, salt, pepper, basil and cook for 10 minutes on high heat.

Serve hot with basil on top.

Spinach and potato soup

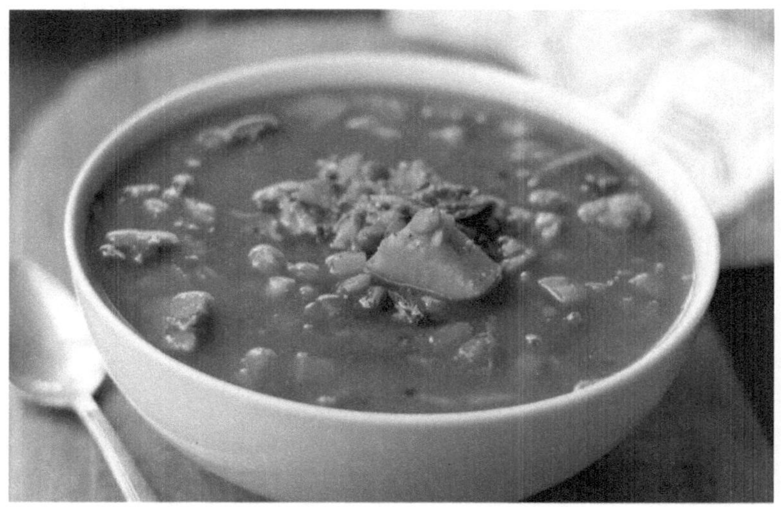

Spinach is very good for our health. But we do not always enjoy eating spinach in salads. Try to spice things up by making a delicious spinach and potato soup. I have used heavy cream here to add more thickness and flavors.

Serving size: 2

Cooking Time: 30 minutes

Ingredients:

- 1 cup heavy cream
- 1 tsp butter
- 1 tsp chopped lemongrass
- 4 leeks, chopped
- 2 cloves garlic, minced
- 2 cup vegetable broth
- 1 cup diced potatoes
- 1 tsp white pepper
- Salt to taste
- 2 cup spinach

Instructions:

Add the spinach in a blender. Blend into a smooth paste.

In a pot melt the butter and toss the potatoes for 1 minute.

Add the lemongrass, leeks, garlic and toss for another minute.

Pour in the broth and cover with lid.

Cook for 15 minutes. Add the heavy cream, spinach paste, salt and pepper.

Cook for another 10 minutes.

Serve hot.

Thick kidney bean soup

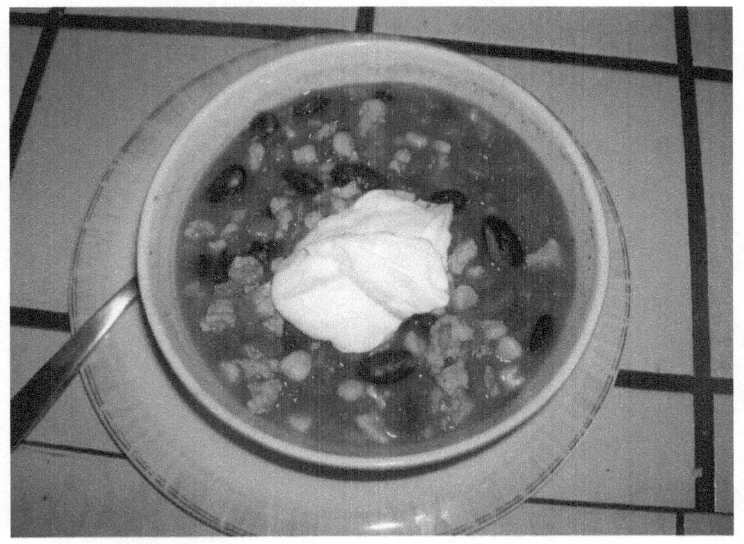

Kidney beans are very good for our health. Kidney bean chili is something everyone loves but kidney bean soup is something that takes less effort and yet tastes good. Whenever I want to make things hassle free in the kitchen, I go for this recipe.

Serving size: 2

Cooking Time: 1 hour

Ingredients:

- 1 cup black bean
- 1 tbsp soy sauce
- 1 tsp garlic paste
- 1 cup tomato paste
- Salt to taste
- Black pepper to taste

Instructions:

Soak the beans in water overnight.

Rinse well and wash them finely.

In an instant pot, add all the ingredients.

Cover with lid. Cook on medium heat for 1 hour.

Serve hot.

Creamy Salmon Curry

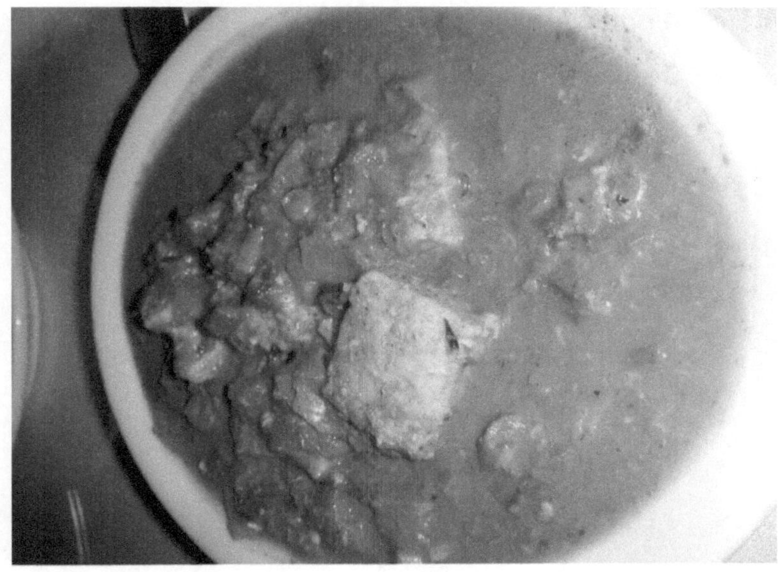

This salmon curry is definitely a restaurant quality meal. It can only 30 minutes to prepare this wonderful dish. The sundried tomatoes adds amazing flavor to this dish.

Serving Size: 4

Cooking Time: 30 minutes

Ingredients:

- ½ cup sun-dried tomatoes
- 4 salmon fillets
- 2 tablespoons olive oil
- 1 teaspoon garlic powder
- 2 onion, chopped
- 1/3 cup chopped spinach
- 1 teaspoon Italian seasoning
- 3 garlic cloves, minced
- 1 cup heavy cream
- ½ cup broth
- 1 cup coconut milk
- ½ cup parmesan cheese

Instructions:

In a large skillet, heat the oil.

Fry the onion, and minced garlic golden brown.

Add the coconut milk, broth, Italian seasoning.

Add the sundried tomatoes and cook on low heat for 10 minutes.

Add the heavy cream, salt and pepper. Cook for 5 minutes.

Add the fish fillet, spinach and cook for another 10 minutes.

Add the parmesan on top and cook until it melts. Serve hot.

Pasta Salad

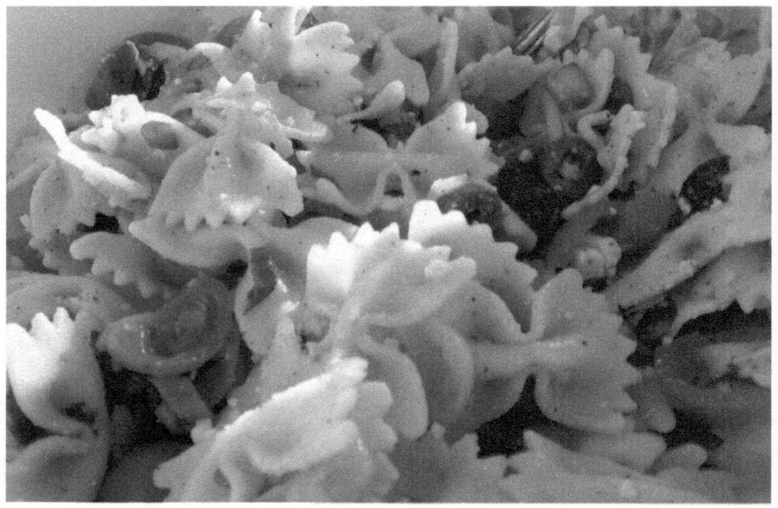

Who does not love pasta? When you want to make pasta healthy, you go for a pasta salad. I have used my favorite vegetables like black olives, green peas, carrots and spinach. You can add any veggie of your choice.

Serving Size: 2

Cooking Time: 10 minutes

Ingredients:

- 1 cup bowtie pasta
- 1/2 cup grated parmesan cheese
- ½ can sun-dried tomatoes
- 1/3 cup green peas
- Salt and pepper to taste
- 1 red bell pepper, diced
- 1 carrot, diced
- ½ cup chopped spinach
- ¼ cup chopped black olives
- 1 tbsp olive oil
- 2 tablespoons white vinegar
- 1/4 cup basil chopped
- 1 tsp mixed herbs

Instructions:

In a pot add 2 cup of water.

Add the pasta and bring it to boil.

Once it is tender, drain well and wash with cold water.

Add into a mixing bowl.

Add all the veggies, herbs, spices into the bowl.

Add the oil, vinegar and mix well. Add salt and pepper and toss again.

Serve cold or fresh.

Pan Fried Chicken Lemon

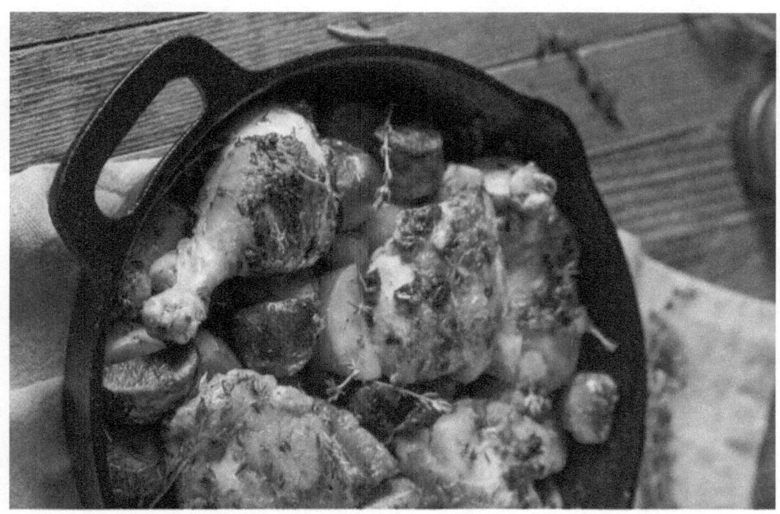

Serving size: 2

Cooking Time: 15 minutes

Ingredients:

- 2 chicken breasts
- 1 Tablespoon butter
- 1 lime, cut into thin slices
- ½ cup chopped basil
- 1 large onion, diced
- 1 tsp tomato sauce
- 1 tsp soy sauce
- ¼ cup grated parmesan cheese
- ½ teaspoon salt
- ¼ teaspoon pepper

Instructions:

In a pan sear the chicken from both sides.

Cut the chicken into small cubes.

In the same pan melt the butter.

Fry the onion golden brown.

Add the tomato sauce, soy sauce, salt, pepper, lime slices and the chicken pieces.

Keep stirring for 5 minutes.

Add the basil and the cheese. Cook for another 4 minutes.

Serve hot with rice.

Grilled Salmon with Peach Salsa

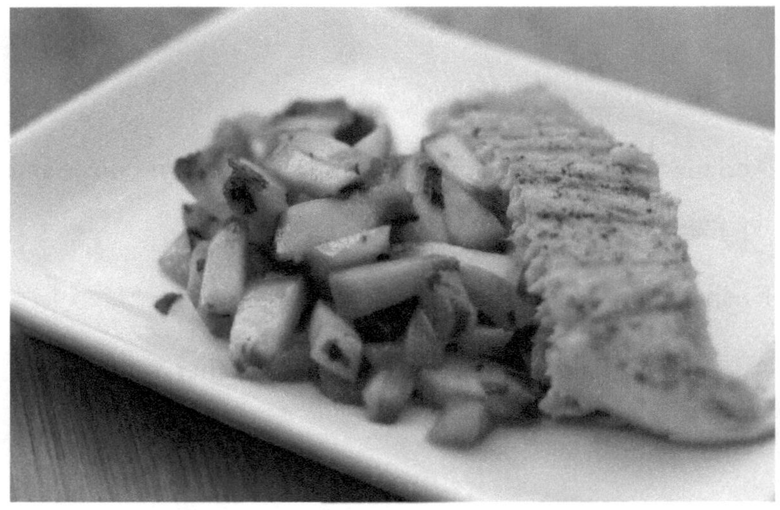

Salmon is very good for us and especially for the expecting mothers! I have combined grilled salmon with a fruity salsa.

Serving Size: 1

Cooking Time: 5 minutes

Ingredients:

- 1 salmon fillet
- 1 avocado, cubed
- 1 apple, cubed
- Fresh coriander, chopped
- Salt and pepper to taste
- 1 tsp tahini paste
- 1 peach, sliced
- 1 red onion, diced

Instructions:

Season the fish with salt and pepper.

Grill the fish to your desired texture.

Transfer to a serving plate.

In a mixing bowl combine the fruits, onion, herb and tahini.

Serve both together.

Zucchini Shrimp Sausage Stir Fry

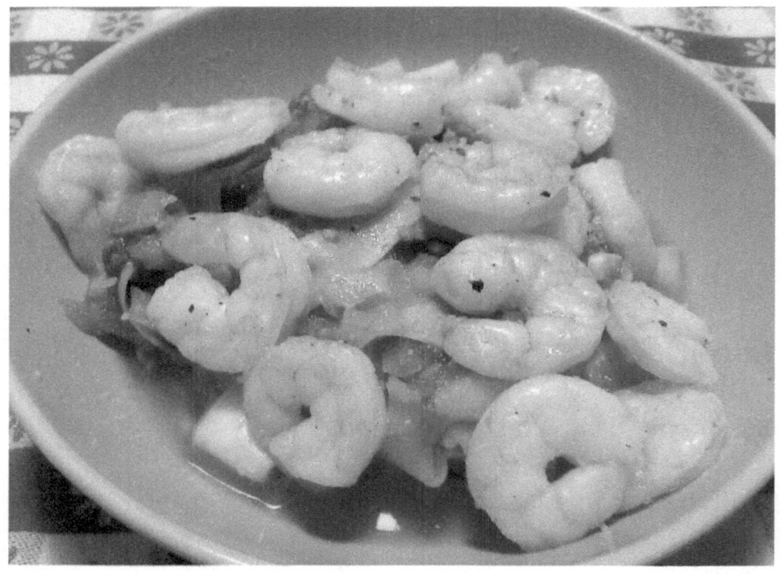

I love to combine protein with veggies. This adds a lot of texture to the dish. I have used veggies like zucchini, squash and asparagus in it. You can add carrots, bell pepper to it too.

Serving Size: 3-4

Cooking Time: 10 minutes

Ingredients:

- 1 lb. shrimp
- 2 Tablespoons butter
- 1 lb. chicken sausage, sliced
- 2 zucchini, sliced
- 1/2 bunch asparagus, diced
- 2 yellow squash, sliced
- 2 Tablespoons mixed herbs
- 1 tsp soy sauce
- Salt and Pepper to taste
- 1 tsp vinegar

Instructions:

Devein the shrimps. Keep the tail intact but remove the skin of the shrimp body.

Melt the butter in a large skillet.

Add the shrimp and fry them for 2 minutes.

Add the rest of the ingredients.

Stir for about 8 minutes. Serve hot.

Chicken in Coconut cream

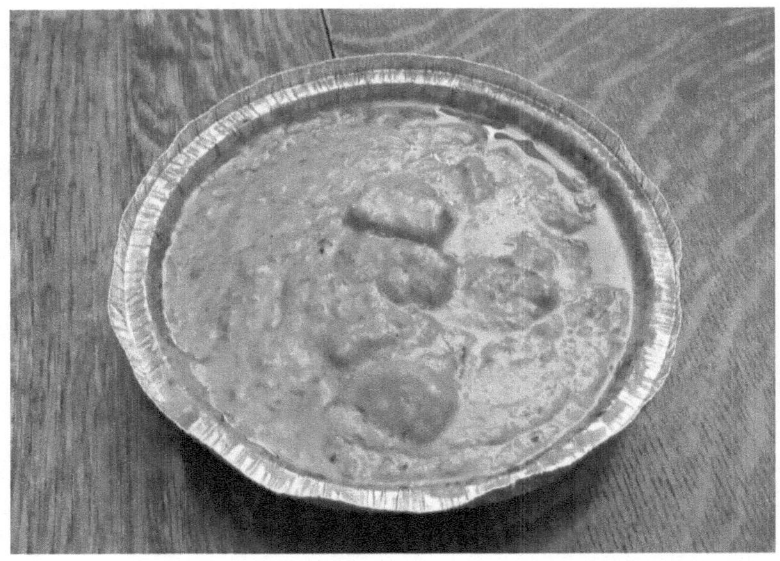

Creamy chicken is such a delicious dish everyone loves. It has a delicious soft texture and it takes very little ingredients and preparation to make it.

Serving size: 2

Cooking Time: 15 minutes

Ingredients:

- 2 chicken breasts
- 2 tbsp butter
- ½ cup coconut cream
- ½ tsp garlic paste
- ½ tsp ginger paste
- ½ tsp onion paste
- Sea salt to taste

Instructions:

Melt the butter in a large pan.

Add the ginger, garlic and onion paste.

Toss for 1 minute and add the chicken.

Let it cook for about 4-5 minutes with low flame.

Add the heavy cream, salt and pepper.

Cook for another 10 minutes.

Serve hot.

Chicken Papaya curry

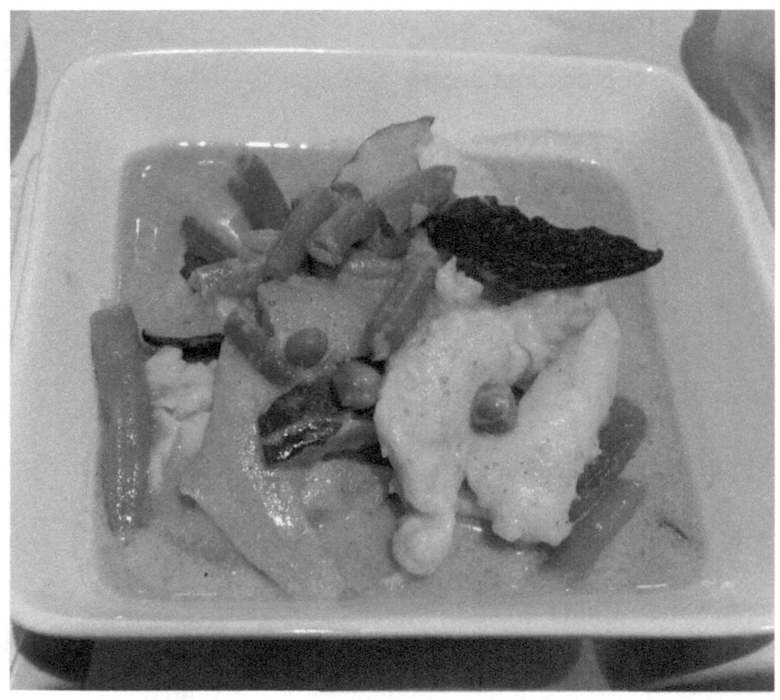

Have you ever heard of this papaya and chicken curry combination! This may sound weird at first but it actually contains a lot of flavors. Papaya is good for digestion, so very good during pregnancy.

Serving size: 4

Cooking Time: 30 minutes

Ingredients:

- 1 lb. chicken
- 1 cup onion, diced
- 1 lb. papaya, cut in bite size pieces
- 1 cup chicken broth
- 2 tbsp olive oil
- 4 green chilies cut in half
- 1 tsp cumin powder
- ½ tsp turmeric powder
- 1 tsp garlic paste
- Salt and pepper to taste

Instructions:

Discard the skin of the chicken. Discard the intestines. Cut the chicken into 8 pieces.

In a pot heat the oil.

Fry the papaya golden brown and transfer to a plate.

In the same pan fry the chicken golden brown and transfer to a plate.

Add the ginger paste, onion, all the spices and the broth.

Cover and cook for 5 minutes.

Return the chicken to the pot and cook for 10 minutes.

Add the salt, chilies, pepper and cook for 2 minutes.

Add the papaya and cook for another 5 minutes.

Serve hot.

Chicken curry with potato

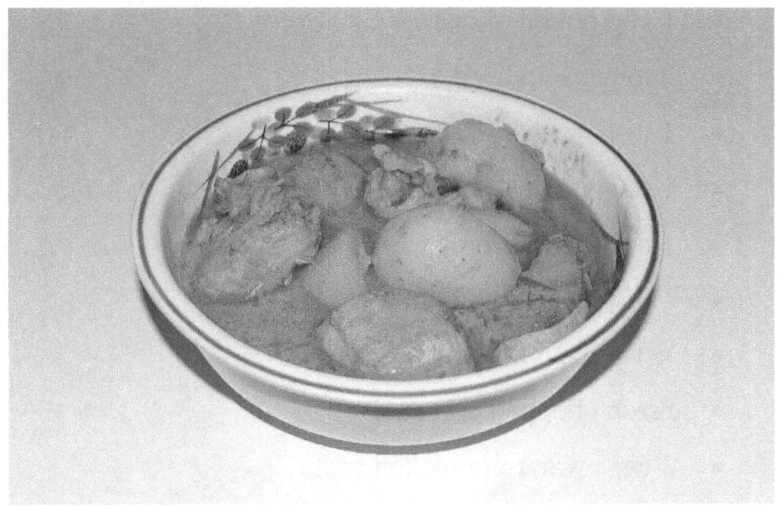

During pregnancy you need to always keep yourself well fed as you are eating for two! This curry is a good way to consume adequate protein and carbohydrate in one dish.

Serving size: 2

Cooking Time: 30 minutes

Ingredients:

- 1 lb. chicken, cut into pieces
- 1 cup potato, diced
- 2 tomatoes, diced
- 1 tbsp ginger paste
- 1 onion, sliced
- 1 tsp turmeric powder
- 1 tbsp garlic paste
- ½ tsp red chili powder
- Fresh chopped coriander
- 2 cups water or chicken broth
- 1 cinnamon stick
- 1 cardamom
- 1 bay leaf
- 4 tbsp mustard oil
- Salt to taste
- 1 tsp coriander powder

Instructions:

Heat the mustard oil in a large pan.

Fry the potatoes golden brown. Transfer to a kitchen towel.

Fry the chicken pieces golden brown and transfer onto a kitchen towel.

Add the onion and fry for 1 minute.

Add the garlic, ginger paste, cinnamon stick, cardamom and bay leaf.

Pour in some water. Let it cook for 4 minutes.

Add the chicken, potato and tomatoes.

Cook for 5 minutes. Add the water or broth.

Add the salt. Cook for about 15 minutes on high heat.

Add the coriander on top and serve hot with rice or tortilla.

Conclusion

When you are eating for two, you always need to be a bit extra careful of what you are eating. This book is dedicated to all the pregnant women who want to eat healthy and delicious food at the same time. These recipes are not too complicated. Some of them are very quick to make and some require a longer time to make. All the recipes are healthy and very much beneficial for an expecting mother. Try these recipes and enjoy a healthy pregnancy journey.

Author's Afterthoughts

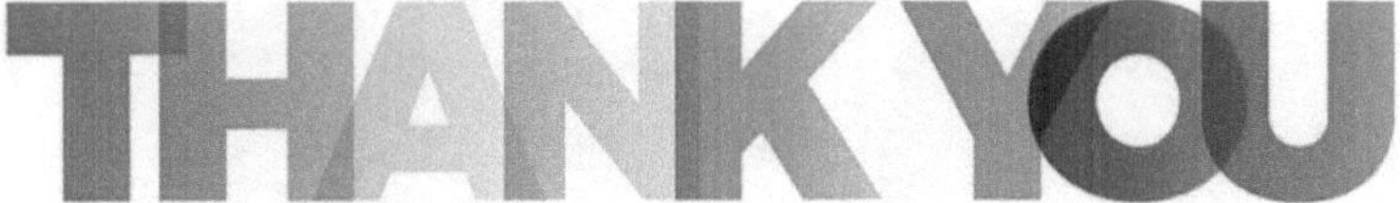

Thanks ever so much to each of my cherished readers for investing the time to read this book!

I know you could have picked from many other books, but you chose this one. So, a big thanks for downloading this book and reading all the way to the end.

If you enjoyed this book or received value from it, I'd like to ask you for a favor. Please take a few minutes to post an honest and heartfelt review on Amazon.com. Your support does make a difference and helps to benefit other people.

Thanks for your Reviews!

Rachael Rayner

About the Author

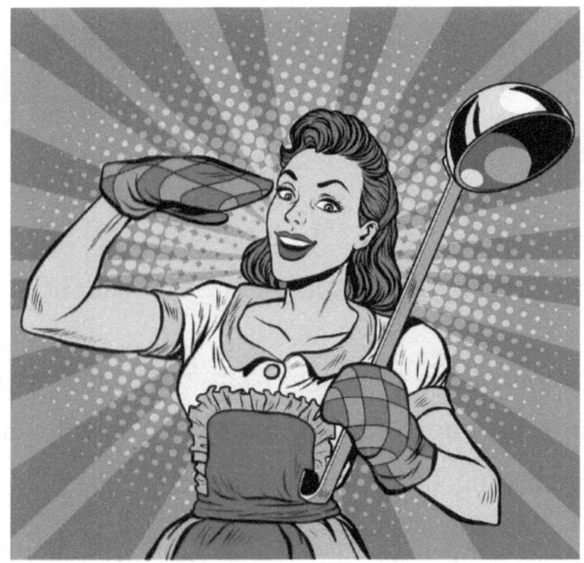

Rachael Rayner

Are you tired of cooking the same types of dishes over and over again? As a mother of not one, but two sets of twins, preparing meals became very challenging, very early on. Not only was it difficult to get enough time in the kitchen to prepare anything other than fried eggs, but I was constantly trying to please 4 little hungry mouths under 5 years old. Of course I would not trade my angels for anything in the world, but I had just about given up on cooking, when I had a genius idea one afternoon while I was napping beside one of my sons. I am so happy and proud to tell you that since then, my kitchen has become my sanctuary and my children have become my helpers. I have transformed my meal preparation, my grocery shopping habits, and my cooking style. I am Racheal Rayner, and I am proud to tell you that I am no longer the boring mom sous-chef people avoid. I am the house in our neighborhood where every kid (and parent) wants to come for dinner.

I was raised Jewish in a very traditional household, and I was not allowed in the kitchen that much. My mother cooked the same recipes day in day out, and salt and pepper were probably the extent of the seasonings we were able to detect in the dishes she made. We did not even know any better until we moved out of the house. My husband, Frank is a foodie. I thought I was too, until I met him. I mean I love food, but who doesn't right? He revolutionized my knowledge about cooking. He used to take over in the kitchen, because after all, we were a modern couple and both of us worked full time jobs. He prepared chilies, soups, chicken casseroles—one more delicious than the last. When I got pregnant with my first set of twins and had to stay home on bed rest, I took over the kitchen and it was a disaster. I tried so hard to find the right ingredients and recipes to make the dishes taste something close to my husband's. However, I hated follow recipes. You don't tell a pregnant woman that her food tastes bad, so Frank and I reluctantly ate the dishes I prepared on week days. Fortunately, he was the weekend chef.

After the birth of my first set of twins, I was too busy to even attempt to cook. Sure, I prepared thousands of bottles of milk and purees, but Frank and I ended up eating take out 4 days out of 5. Then, no break for this mom, I gave birth to my second set of twins only 19 months later! I knew that now it was not just about Frank and I anymore, but it was about these little ones for whom I wanted to cook healthy meals, and I had to learn how to cook.

One afternoon in March, when I got up from that power nap with my boys, I had figured out what I needed to do to improve my cooking skills and stop torturing my family with my bland dishes. I had to let go of everything I had learned, tasted, or seen from my childhood and start over. I spent a week organizing my kitchen, and I equipped myself a new blender. I also got some fun shaped cookie cutters, a rolling pin, wooden spatulas, mixing bowls, fruit cutters, and plenty of plastic storage containers. I was ready.

My oldest twins, Isabella and Sophia are now teenagers, and love to cook with their Mom when they are not too busy talking on the phone. My youngest twins Erick and John, are now 10 years old and so helpful in the kitchen, especially when it's time to make cookies.

Let me start sharing my tips, recipes, and shopping suggestions with you ladies and gentlemen. I did not reinvent the wheel here but I did make my kitchen my own, started storing my favorite baking ingredients, and visiting the fresh produce market more often. I have mastered the principles of slow cooking and chopping veggies ahead of time. I have even embraced the involvement of my little ones in the kitchen with me.

I never want to hear you say that you are too busy to cook some delicious and healthy dishes, because BUSY, is my middle name.